Rice Flour Guide for Beginners

Nutritional Value of Rice Flour

By

Darian Jamie

Table of Contents

CHAPTER 1

Introduction

Rice flour, a versatile and gluten-free alternative to traditional wheat flour, has become an integral component of modern cooking. Its significance goes beyond mere substitution, contributing unique textures, flavors, and nutritional attributes to a myriad of culinary creations.

1.1 Importance of Rice Flour in Cooking

The importance of rice flour in cooking transcends its gluten-free nature, addressing the dietary needs of individuals with gluten sensitivities or those adhering to a gluten-free lifestyle. As a staple in many Asian cuisines, rice flour serves as the foundation for a multitude of dishes, ranging from delectable desserts to savory delicacies. Its neutral taste and fine texture make it an adaptable ingredient, seamlessly blending into recipes and enhancing the overall culinary experience.

Beyond its practical applications, rice flour brings a unique set of attributes to the table. It is a key player in gluten-free baking, providing structure and moisture retention in the absence of gluten. This makes it an essential component for those seeking to create light and fluffy cakes, cookies, and bread without compromising on taste and texture. Moreover, rice flour serves as an excellent thickening agent in soups, sauces, and gravies, offering a gluten-free alternative to conventional wheat-based thickeners.

1.2 Overview of Rice Flour Varieties

Rice flour is not a one-size-fits-all ingredient; rather, it encompasses a spectrum of varieties, each with its distinct characteristics. Understanding these variations is crucial for achieving the desired results in different culinary endeavors.

- **White Rice Flour:** Refined from polished white rice, this flour has a mild flavor and fine texture. It is commonly used in baking and as a thickening agent.

- **Brown Rice Flour:** Derived from whole brown rice, this

variety retains the bran and germ, imparting a nuttier flavor and coarser texture. Brown rice flour is often favored for its increased nutritional content.

- **Sweet Rice Flour (Glutinous Rice Flour):** Despite its name, sweet rice flour is gluten-free. It is known for its sticky texture, making it an ideal choice for gluten-free pastries, dumplings, and Asian desserts.

- **Rice Starch:** Extracted from rice, this starch is used primarily as a thickening agent in sauces and puddings. Its neutral taste and translucent appearance make it a versatile choice in culinary applications.

- **Rice Bran Powder:** Incorporating the nutrient-rich

outer layer of rice, this variety adds a nutritional boost to recipes. Its slightly coarse texture makes it suitable for use in certain baked goods and coatings.

As we navigate the diverse landscape of rice flour varieties, it becomes evident that each type brings its own nuances to the culinary canvas, allowing chefs and home cooks alike to tailor their creations to specific preferences and dietary requirements.

CHAPTER 2

Understanding Rice Flour

2.1 What is Rice Flour?

Rice flour, a fundamental ingredient in many culinary traditions, is a finely milled powder derived from rice grains. The production process involves milling rice to remove the outer layers, resulting in a versatile, gluten-free flour. The transformation of rice into flour unlocks a myriad of culinary possibilities, allowing it to serve as a foundation for an array of dishes, both sweet and savory.

One of the defining features of rice flour is its absence of gluten, making it an indispensable resource for individuals with gluten sensitivities or those adhering to a gluten-free diet. The neutral flavor and fine texture of rice flour make it an adaptable ingredient, seamlessly integrating into recipes without overpowering other elements. Its application extends across various cuisines, contributing to the creation of baked goods, pastries, noodles, and a multitude of other culinary delights.

As we navigate the realm of rice flour, it is essential to recognize that the absence of gluten necessitates distinct considerations in cooking and baking. Understanding how rice flour interacts with other ingredients, as well as its unique characteristics, empowers chefs to create culinary masterpieces that cater to a diverse range of dietary preferences.

2.2 Types of Rice Used in Rice Flour

The type of rice utilized in the production of rice flour significantly influences its flavor, texture, and nutritional content. Different varieties of rice impart distinct qualities to the resulting flour, allowing for a spectrum of choices to cater to specific culinary needs.

- **Short-Grain Rice:** This type of rice, known for its plump and almost round grains, is commonly used to produce rice flour. Short-grain rice contributes to a flour with a slightly moister texture, making it particularly suitable for certain types of baking, such as in the creation of Japanese mochi or rice cakes.

- **Long-Grain Rice:** With its elongated grains, long-grain rice yields a flour with a lighter and fluffier texture. This variety is often preferred in gluten-free baking, providing a delicate crumb structure in cakes and cookies.

- **Medium-Grain Rice:** Falling between short and long-grain varieties, medium-grain rice produces a flour that strikes a balance in texture. It is versatile and can be used in a variety of recipes, including both sweet and savory dishes.

- **Specialty Rice:** Varieties such as glutinous rice (sticky rice) and aromatic rice (such as Jasmine or Basmati) offer unique flavor profiles and textures to rice flour. Glutinous rice flour, despite its name, is gluten-free and is prized for its sticky consistency, making it ideal for certain Asian desserts and dumplings.

Understanding the nuances of these rice varieties provides chefs and home cooks with the knowledge to select the most suitable rice flour for their specific culinary endeavors. Whether pursuing a chewy texture in a dessert or a light and airy crumb in a cake, the choice of rice plays a pivotal role in achieving the desired outcome.

2.3 Nutritional Value of Rice Flour

Beyond its culinary versatility and gluten-free attributes, rice flour brings a wealth of nutritional value to the table. Understanding the nutritional composition of rice flour is essential for those seeking not only delicious but also health-conscious culinary choices.

- **Carbohydrates:** Rice flour is primarily composed of carbohydrates, providing a significant source of energy. The complex carbohydrates in rice flour contribute to sustained energy release, making it a suitable choice for those looking to maintain stable blood sugar levels.

- **Protein:** While rice flour is not as protein-dense as some other flours, it still contributes a modest amount of protein to recipes. Protein is crucial for various bodily functions, including the repair and maintenance of tissues.

- **Dietary Fiber:** Depending on the type of rice used, rice flour can contain dietary fiber. Brown rice flour, in particular, retains more fiber as it includes the bran and germ of the rice. Dietary fiber is essential for digestive health and can contribute to a feeling of fullness.

- **Vitamins and Minerals:** Rice flour contains various vitamins and minerals, including B vitamins (such as B1, B2, and B3), iron, and magnesium. These nutrients play vital roles in energy metabolism, red blood cell formation, and overall immune function.

- **Low in Fat:** Rice flour is naturally low in fat, making it a suitable choice for those looking to reduce their fat intake. This characteristic makes it an attractive option for individuals aiming for a well-balanced and low-fat diet.

- **Gluten-Free:** Perhaps one of the most significant nutritional aspects of rice flour is its gluten-free nature. For individuals with celiac disease or gluten sensitivities, rice flour provides a safe alternative, allowing them to enjoy a variety of dishes without compromising their dietary restrictions.

It's important to note that the nutritional content can vary depending on the type of rice used to produce the flour. Brown rice flour, for instance, retains more nutrients compared to white rice flour due to the inclusion of the rice bran and germ.

Incorporating rice flour into a well-balanced diet offers not only a versatile culinary experience but also nutritional benefits. Chefs and home cooks can harness the nutritional richness of rice flour to create meals that are not only delicious but also contribute to overall health and well-being.

CHAPTER 3

How is Rice Flour Made?

The journey from whole rice grains to the fine powder that is rice flour involves intricate processes that have evolved over time.

3.1 Traditional Milling Processes

Traditional methods of producing rice flour are deeply rooted in cultural practices and often involve time-honored techniques passed down through generations. The process typically unfolds as follows:

- **Harvesting and Drying:** The first step involves harvesting mature rice plants and allowing the rice grains to dry thoroughly. Proper drying is crucial for achieving the desired texture in the final product.

- **Hulling:** Once dried, the rice undergoes hulling, a process where the outer husk is removed from the grains. This can be done manually or using traditional tools such as grinding stones or wooden pestles.

- **Milling:** After hulling, the rice is milled to remove the bran layers, resulting in white rice. The milling process can be accomplished using hand-operated mills or community mills, where rice is ground into a coarse powder.

- **Finer Milling for Flour:** For rice flour, the milled white rice undergoes further grinding to achieve a finer texture. This step is critical for obtaining the desired consistency in the final product.

- **Sifting:** Traditional methods often involve sifting the ground rice to separate the finer flour from coarser particles. This manual process helps refine the texture of the rice flour.

Traditional milling processes are labor-intensive and time-consuming, reflecting the craftsmanship embedded in traditional culinary practices. While these methods hold cultural significance, advancements in technology have given rise to more efficient and scalable approaches.

3.2 Modern Rice Flour Production

Modern industrial processes have streamlined the production of rice flour, making it more accessible on a larger scale. The steps involved in modern rice flour production include:

- **Cleaning and Sorting:** Harvested rice undergoes thorough cleaning to remove impurities and foreign particles. The rice is then sorted to ensure uniform quality.

- **Milling:** High-speed milling machines are employed to remove the outer layers of the rice, producing white rice. The milling process is carefully controlled to achieve the desired texture and fineness.

- **Grinding:** The milled white rice is further ground into a fine powder using specialized grinding equipment. This process ensures a consistent particle size, contributing to the uniformity of the final product.

- **Screening and Sifting:** Modern facilities use advanced screening and sifting technologies to separate the finer rice flour from coarser particles. This automation enhances efficiency and precision in the production process.

- **Packaging:** The final step involves packaging the rice

flour into various formats for distribution. Modern packaging technologies help maintain the freshness and quality of the product.

Modern rice flour production benefits from technological advancements, enabling large-scale manufacturing while maintaining quality standards. The efficiency of these processes has contributed to the widespread availability of rice flour in markets worldwide, meeting the demands of diverse culinary preferences and dietary needs.

Understanding the journey from whole rice grains to the refined powder of rice flour provides insight into the craftsmanship and technological innovations that have shaped this essential culinary ingredient.

3.3 Homemade Rice Flour

While commercial rice flour is readily available, crafting rice flour at home offers a unique experience and allows for greater control over the final product's characteristics. Homemade rice flour can be a rewarding venture, especially for those who enjoy the process of creating ingredients from scratch. Here's a step-by-step guide on how to make rice flour at home:

Ingredients and Equipment:

- Raw rice (any variety, such as short-grain, long-grain, or brown rice)

- Blender or food processor

- Fine mesh sieve or flour sifter

- A clean, dry bowl

- Airtight storage container

Procedure:

1. **Choose the Right Rice:** Select the type of rice based on your preferences. Different rice varieties will yield slightly different textures and flavors in the resulting flour. Brown rice, for instance, will provide a nuttier flavor and higher nutritional content due to its retained bran and germ.

2. **Rinse the Rice:** Thoroughly rinse the rice under cold water to remove excess starch. This helps prevent the rice flour from becoming overly sticky during the milling process.

3. **Soak the Rice (Optional):** For a smoother texture, you can soak the rice in water for a few hours or overnight. This step

softens the rice, making it easier to grind.

4. **Drain the Rice:** If you soaked the rice, drain it well to remove excess water.

5. **Grind the Rice:** Place the rice in a blender or food processor. Grind the rice in batches until it reaches a fine powder consistency. This may take several minutes, depending on the power of your equipment.

6. **Sift the Flour:** To achieve a smoother texture, sift the freshly ground rice flour through a fine mesh sieve or flour sifter. This helps separate the finer flour from any remaining coarse particles.

7. **Repeat if Necessary:** If there are still coarse particles after

the first sifting, you can re-grind them and sift again until you achieve the desired consistency.

8. **Store the Rice Flour:** Transfer the homemade rice flour to a clean, dry bowl, and store it in an airtight container. Proper storage helps maintain the freshness and quality of the flour.

Tips:

- Ensure that both the rice and equipment are dry, as moisture can affect the texture of the flour.

- Experiment with different rice varieties to discover the flavors and textures that best suit your culinary preferences.

- Adjust the fineness of the flour based on your intended use—finer for delicate pastries and coarser for certain savory dishes.

Crafting rice flour at home allows for customization and a connection to the traditional methods of food preparation. Whether for dietary preferences, experimentation, or the joy of culinary creation, homemade rice flour adds a personal touch to your cooking endeavors.

CHAPTER 4

Using Rice Flour in Cooking

4.1 Baking with Rice Flour

Rice flour's gluten-free nature and versatile texture make it a go-to ingredient for gluten-free baking. Here, we'll explore the broader category of gluten-free baking and how rice flour can be seamlessly integrated into a variety of sweet treats.

4.1.1 Gluten-Free Baking

One of the primary advantages of rice flour is its suitability for those following a gluten-free diet. Gluten, a protein found in wheat and other grains, can cause adverse reactions in individuals with celiac disease or gluten sensitivities. Rice flour steps in as an excellent alternative, offering a light and tender texture to gluten-free baked goods.

- **Gluten-Free Cakes and Cupcakes:** Rice flour can be used as the primary flour in gluten-free cake and cupcake recipes. Its fine texture contributes to a delicate crumb, and the neutral flavor allows other ingredients to shine.

- **Cookies and Bars:** Incorporating rice flour into gluten-free cookie and bar recipes results in treats with a satisfying texture. It helps maintain the structure and moisture content without the need for gluten.

- **Pancakes and Waffles:** For a gluten-free breakfast, rice flour can be used to create light and fluffy pancakes or crisp waffles. Its ability to mimic the properties of traditional flour makes it a versatile choice for breakfast delights.

- **Gluten-Free Pastries:** Whether crafting gluten-free pie crusts or puff pastry, rice flour can be part of a blend that provides the desired flakiness and texture.

When embarking on gluten-free baking with rice flour, it's often beneficial to combine it with other gluten-free flours or starches, such as tapioca flour or potato starch, to achieve the best results. Experimenting with different ratios allows for the development of recipes that suit individual taste preferences.

4.1.2 Substituting Rice Flour for All-Purpose Flour

Rice flour's adaptability extends beyond gluten-free baking, making it a suitable substitute for all-purpose flour in various recipes. Here are some considerations when substituting rice flour for all-purpose flour:

- **1:1 Substitution:** In many recipes, you can replace all-purpose flour with an equal amount of rice flour. This is particularly effective in recipes where a lighter texture is desirable, such as in certain cakes and cookies.

- **Texture Adjustments:** Rice flour has a different texture than all-purpose flour, which can affect the final product. In some cases, you may need to adjust the quantities or combine rice flour with other flours to achieve the desired texture.

- **Binding Agents:** Since rice flour lacks gluten, incorporating binding agents such as xanthan gum or guar gum may be necessary, especially in recipes that rely on gluten for structure.

- **Bread and Yeast-Based Recipes:** When substituting rice flour for all-purpose flour in bread or other yeast-based recipes, additional considerations may be needed. Adding vital wheat gluten or using a blend of rice flour with other gluten-free flours can

help mimic the elasticity
provided by gluten.

Experimenting with different recipes and keeping track of adjustments allows for the development of a personalized approach to substituting rice flour for all-purpose flour. Whether aiming for gluten-free options or simply exploring new textures and flavors, rice flour provides a versatile canvas for culinary creativity.

4.2 Cooking Savory Dishes with Rice Flour

While rice flour is often celebrated for its role in sweet treats, its versatility extends to savory dishes as well. In this section, we'll explore how rice flour can be a valuable ingredient in enhancing the texture and flavor of various savory creations.

4.2.1 Thickening Agents in Soups and Sauces

Rice flour's ability to act as a thickening agent makes it an excellent choice for soups, stews, and sauces. Whether you're aiming to achieve a velvety consistency or adapt a recipe to be gluten-free, rice flour can be a valuable addition to your culinary toolkit.

- **Roux Replacement:** In traditional cooking, a roux (a mixture of flour and fat) is often used to thicken soups and sauces. For a gluten-free alternative, rice flour can be employed in a similar manner. Simply whisk rice flour into melted butter or oil to create a gluten-free roux.

- **Sauce Thickening:** When preparing sauces, rice flour can be added directly to the liquid to create a smooth and lump-free consistency. This is particularly useful in recipes where a lighter texture is desired.

- **Gluten-Free Gravies:** Rice flour can be the key to crafting rich and flavorful gluten-free gravies. Whether accompanying roasted meats or mashed potatoes, the addition of rice flour ensures a satisfying thickness.

When using rice flour as a thickening agent, it's essential to mix it with a small amount of cold liquid before incorporating it into the hot mixture. This prevents lumps from forming and ensures even distribution.

4.2.2 Coating for Frying

Rice flour's unique properties make it an excellent choice for creating crispy and light coatings in frying. Whether you're preparing tempura, fried chicken, or vegetables, rice flour can contribute to a delightful crunch.

- **Tempura Batter:** Rice flour is a key ingredient in tempura batter, a Japanese technique that results in a light and airy coating for vegetables, seafood, or meats. The absence of gluten in rice flour allows the batter to stay delicate and crisp.

- **Fried Chicken Coating:** When used in combination with other seasonings, rice flour can be an exceptional coating for fried chicken. It creates a thin, crispy layer that enhances the overall texture of the dish.

- **Vegetable Fritters:** Rice flour can be incorporated into batters for vegetable fritters or pakoras, providing a crisp exterior while allowing the natural flavors of the vegetables to shine.

In addition to its texture-enhancing qualities, rice flour's neutral flavor ensures that it won't overpower the taste of the ingredients it coats. The lightness it imparts makes it an ideal choice for achieving that sought-after crispy texture.

CHAPTER 5

Tips for Storing Rice Flour

Proper storage is crucial to maintaining the freshness, quality, and usability of rice flour over time. Here are some tips to ensure that your rice flour remains in optimal condition:

5.1 Shelf Life of Rice Flour

The shelf life of rice flour can vary based on factors such as the type of rice used, the milling process, and storage conditions. Here are some general guidelines to help you understand and maximize the shelf life of your rice flour:

- **Check the Expiry Date:** If you purchase commercially packaged rice flour, be sure to check the expiry or "best by" date on the packaging. This date provides an indication of the manufacturer's recommended timeframe for optimal quality.

- **Store in a Cool, Dry Place:** Rice flour, like many flours, is susceptible to moisture. To prevent clumping and the development of mold, store rice flour in a cool, dry place. Consider transferring it to an airtight container to protect it from humidity and odors.

- **Avoid Sunlight and Heat:**
Exposure to sunlight and heat
can lead to the deterioration of
rice flour. Store it away from
direct sunlight and heat
sources, such as stovetops or
ovens.

- **Use a Sealed Container:** Air
can contribute to the
degradation of rice flour over
time. Keep it in a sealed,
airtight container to minimize
exposure to air and maintain
freshness. This is particularly
important if you buy rice flour
in larger quantities.

- **Label the Storage Container:**
If you transfer rice flour to a
different container, label it with
the date of purchase or the date
you opened the original

packaging. This helps you keep track of its freshness.

- **Refrigeration or Freezing (Optional):** While rice flour doesn't require refrigeration, storing it in the refrigerator or freezer can extend its shelf life. If you choose this option, ensure the flour is in a moisture-proof container to prevent condensation upon thawing.

- **Perform a Quality Check:** Periodically check the rice flour for any signs of spoilage, such as off odors, discoloration, or the presence of insects. If you notice any of these signs, it's advisable to discard the flour.

By following these storage tips, you can prolong the shelf life of your rice flour and ensure that it maintains its quality for an extended period. Proper storage not only preserves the flour's texture and flavor but also contributes to the success of your culinary endeavors when using rice flour in various recipes.

5.2 Proper Storage Conditions for Rice Flour

Ensuring the proper storage conditions for rice flour is essential to maintain its freshness, prevent spoilage, and preserve its quality. Here are specific guidelines on how to store rice flour effectively:

1. **Use Airtight Containers:** Transfer your rice flour from its original packaging to a clean, airtight container. A sealed container helps prevent

exposure to air, which can lead to oxidation and the development of off flavors.

2. **Choose a Cool and Dry Location:** Store rice flour in a cool, dry place, away from direct sunlight and heat sources. Excessive heat can accelerate the deterioration of the flour, while humidity can lead to clumping and spoilage. A pantry or cupboard is an ideal location.

3. **Avoid Odorous Environments:** Rice flour can absorb odors from its surroundings. Store it away from strong-smelling items such as spices, onions, or cleaning supplies to preserve its natural flavor.

4. **Label the Container:** If you transfer rice flour to a different container, label it with the date of purchase or the date it was opened. This helps you keep track of its freshness and ensures that older flour is used first.

5. **Consider Refrigeration or Freezing (Optional):** While rice flour generally has a long shelf life when stored properly, if you anticipate infrequent use or want to extend its freshness, you can refrigerate or freeze it. Place the flour in a moisture-proof container to prevent condensation. Allow it to come to room temperature before use.

6. **Inspect Regularly:** Periodically check the rice flour for signs of spoilage. If you

notice any unusual odors, discoloration, or the presence of insects, discard the flour. Performing regular inspections ensures that you use high-quality ingredients in your cooking.

7. **Store Different Varieties Separately:** If you have multiple varieties of rice flour, consider storing them separately to maintain their individual characteristics. For example, sweet rice flour (glutinous rice flour) may have different storage needs than regular rice flour.

8. **Rotate Stock:** If you purchase rice flour in larger quantities, practice stock rotation. Use older batches first to ensure that your supply remains fresh.

9. **Repackage if Necessary:** If your rice flour comes in packaging that is not airtight, or if the packaging is damaged, consider repackaging it in an airtight container to maintain its quality.

Adhering to these proper storage conditions, you can maximize the shelf life of your rice flour, ensuring that it remains a reliable and flavorful ingredient for your culinary endeavors. Whether you're using it for gluten-free baking, thickening soups, or creating crispy coatings, well-preserved rice flour enhances the overall success of your recipes.

5.3 Avoiding Contamination of Rice Flour

Preventing contamination is crucial to ensuring the safety and quality of rice flour. Here are key practices to follow to avoid contamination:

1. **Clean Storage Containers:** Before transferring rice flour to a new container, ensure it is clean and free from any residue. Wash containers with mild soap and water, and make sure they are thoroughly dried before use.

2. **Use Clean Utensils:** When measuring or scooping rice flour, use clean and dry utensils. Moisture can contribute to clumping and contamination, so avoid using wet utensils.

3. **Hand Hygiene:** Wash your hands thoroughly before handling rice flour, especially if you are transferring it to a different container or using it in a recipe. Clean hands help prevent the introduction of contaminants.

4. **Seal Containers Properly:** Ensure that storage containers are sealed tightly after each use. This prevents dust, pests, and airborne contaminants from entering and affecting the quality of the rice flour.

5. **Avoid Cross-Contamination:** Be mindful of the surfaces and utensils you use when working with other ingredients, especially those containing allergens. Cross-contamination can occur if traces of allergens

are introduced into the rice
flour, posing risks for
individuals with allergies.

6. **Keep the Storage Area Clean:**
   Regularly clean and maintain
   the storage area for rice flour.
   Wipe down shelves, check for
   signs of pests, and ensure that
   the storage space is free from
   debris or spillages.

7. **Inspect for Pests:** Periodically
   inspect both the rice flour
   container and the storage area
   for any signs of pests, such as
   insects or rodents. If you notice
   any infestation, take immediate
   steps to address the issue and
   consider discarding the affected
   flour.

8. **Store Away from Non-Food
   Items:** Keep rice flour away

from non-food items,
chemicals, or cleaning supplies.
Storing it in a designated food
storage area reduces the risk of
contamination.

9. **Buy from Reputable Sources:**
Choose reputable brands or
suppliers when purchasing rice
flour. This reduces the
likelihood of contamination
during the manufacturing and
packaging processes.

10. **Separate Storage for Different Varieties:** If you
have various types of rice flour,
store them separately to prevent
flavor or aroma transfer
between different varieties.

Following these guidelines, you can
minimize the risk of contamination
and ensure that your rice flour

remains a safe and reliable ingredient for your culinary endeavors. Practicing good hygiene, proper storage, and regular inspections contribute to a clean and well-maintained kitchen environment.

CHAPTER 6

Common Issues and Solutions

In the course of working with rice flour, certain issues may arise that can affect the texture and overall quality of your culinary creations. One common challenge is the tendency of rice flour to clump. Here's how you can prevent and address clumping:

6.1 Preventing Clumping

- **Dry Ingredients:** Begin with ensuring that both the rice flour and any other dry ingredients in your recipe are well sifted and free-flowing. This helps create a smoother texture and minimizes the likelihood of clumps forming when liquids are added.

- **Room Temperature Ingredients:** Make sure that ingredients like eggs and liquids are at room temperature before incorporating them into the rice flour. Cold ingredients can cause the rice flour to clump due to temperature differences.

- **Gradual Liquid Addition:** When adding liquids to rice flour, do so gradually. Pouring

in large amounts at once can
lead to uneven moisture
absorption and the formation of
clumps. Mix consistently while
adding the liquid to encourage a
smooth blend.

- **Use a Whisk or Sifter:**
  Employ a whisk or a sifter to
  combine rice flour with other
  dry ingredients or to
  incorporate liquids. This helps
  break up any potential clumps
  and ensures an even
  distribution of moisture.

- **Room for Rest:** Allow the rice
  flour mixture to rest for a few
  minutes before further
  processing. This brief resting
  period gives the flour particles
  time to absorb the liquid more
  evenly, reducing the likelihood
  of clumping.

- **Adjust Liquid Content:** If you find that your rice flour mixture is too thick and prone to clumping, adjust the liquid content slightly. Conversely, if it's too thin, consider adding a bit more rice flour. Achieving the right consistency is key to preventing clumps.

- **Straining or Sieving:** If clumps have already formed, strain or sieve the mixture to remove them. This can be done before incorporating the rice flour mixture into the larger recipe or directly into the final dish.

- **Consider Flour Blends:** Depending on the recipe, you might explore using a blend of rice flour with other gluten-free flours or starches. This can enhance the texture and reduce the tendency of rice flour to clump.

By being mindful of these preventive measures and employing solutions as needed, you can overcome the challenge of clumping and enjoy the benefits of rice flour in your cooking and baking endeavors. The goal is to achieve a smooth, lump-free consistency that enhances the quality of your dishes.

6.2 Dealing with Grittiness

Another issue that may arise when working with rice flour is the potential for grittiness in the final product. Grittiness can be caused by the coarser particles present in certain types of rice flour. Here are some strategies to address and minimize grittiness:

1. **Choose a Finer Grind:** Opt for a finer grind of rice flour, especially if you are concerned about grittiness. Some commercially available rice flours are labeled as "superfine" or "extra fine," indicating a finer texture.

2. **Sift the Flour:** Before incorporating rice flour into your recipe, sift it to remove any coarse particles. This step helps achieve a smoother consistency and reduces the likelihood of grittiness in the finished product.

3. **Blend with Other Flours:** Consider blending rice flour with other gluten-free flours or

starches. This not only adds complexity to the flavor but can also contribute to a smoother texture. Experiment with different flour combinations to find the blend that works best for your specific recipe.

4. **Soak the Flour:** If the grittiness is a persistent issue, you can try soaking the rice flour in liquid before incorporating it into your recipe. This gives the flour particles time to absorb moisture and may result in a smoother texture.

5. **Use Different Rice Varieties:** Different varieties of rice can produce rice flour with varying textures. Experiment with rice flour made from different rice varieties to find one that aligns

with your preferences for
texture and grittiness.

6. **Adjust Liquid Content:**
Grittiness can sometimes be a
result of insufficient moisture.
Adjust the liquid content in
your recipe, adding a bit more
if needed, to ensure proper
hydration of the rice flour
particles.

7. **Explore Pre-Made Blends:**
Some pre-made gluten-free
flour blends, designed for
specific purposes like baking or
thickening, may already include
a combination of flours to
achieve a smoother texture.
These blends are formulated to
address issues like grittiness.

8. **Cook or Bake Thoroughly:**
Cooking or baking the recipe

thoroughly can sometimes help minimize grittiness. The cooking process allows the rice flour to absorb more moisture and soften, contributing to a smoother texture in the final dish.

Experimenting with these strategies and adjusting your approach based on the specific recipe and desired outcome can help you overcome issues of grittiness when using rice flour. It's important to find the balance that works best for your culinary preferences and the requirements of the dish you're preparing.

6.3 Addressing Moisture-related Problems

Moisture-related issues can arise when working with rice flour, affecting the texture and consistency of your recipes. Here are some strategies to address and prevent common moisture-related problems:

1. **Storage Awareness:**

   - Ensure rice flour is stored in a cool, dry place to prevent moisture absorption.

   - Use airtight containers to protect rice flour from humidity and external moisture.

2. **Prevent Clumping:**

   - Keep all utensils and equipment dry when working with rice flour.

   - Gradually add liquids to rice flour and mix

consistently to prevent clumping.

- Store rice flour away from high-moisture areas in the kitchen.

3. **Adjust Liquid Content:**

   - If a recipe turns out too dry, consider adjusting the liquid content slightly to achieve the desired consistency.

   - Be cautious when adding liquids, doing so gradually to avoid over-hydration.

4. **Use Room Temperature Ingredients:**

   - Ensure that ingredients like eggs and liquids are at room temperature before incorporating them into rice flour recipes. Cold ingredients can affect the overall texture.

5. **Avoid Excessive Moisture in Gluten-Free Baking:**

   - In gluten-free baking, be mindful of the moisture content. Some gluten-free flours, including rice flour, may absorb more moisture than traditional flours.

6. **Blend with Other Flours:**

   - Experiment with blending rice flour with other gluten-free flours or starches to balance moisture absorption and enhance texture.

7. **Consider Binders:**

   - In recipes where the absence of gluten might impact structure, consider adding binders such as xanthan gum or guar gum to help improve texture and prevent excessive moisture absorption.

8. **Check Consistency During Mixing:**

   - Regularly check the consistency of the batter or dough during mixing. Adjust the liquid content or add more rice flour if necessary to achieve the desired consistency.

9. **Strive for Uniform Hydration:**

- Aim for uniform hydration of rice flour particles throughout the mixture. Uneven hydration can lead to a clumpy or uneven texture.

10. **Allow for Resting Periods:**

- Let the rice flour mixture rest for a few minutes before further processing. This allows for even hydration and minimizes the risk of moisture-related issues.

Incorporating these strategies into your cooking and baking practices, you can address and prevent moisture-related problems associated with rice flour. Experimentation and adjustments based on specific recipes and desired outcomes will help you achieve optimal results in your culinary endeavors.

CHAPTER 7

Recipes with Rice Flour

7.1 Gluten-Free Pancakes with Rice Flour

Enjoy light and fluffy pancakes without gluten with this simple and delicious gluten-free pancake recipe featuring rice flour. These pancakes are perfect for a leisurely breakfast or brunch.

Ingredients:

- 1 cup rice flour

- 2 tablespoons sugar

- 1 teaspoon baking powder

- 1/2 teaspoon baking soda

- 1/4 teaspoon salt

- 1 cup buttermilk (or dairy-free alternative)

- 1 large egg

- 2 tablespoons melted butter (or oil for dairy-free option)

- 1 teaspoon vanilla extract

- Additional butter or oil for cooking

Instructions:

1. **Prepare the Dry Ingredients:**

   - In a mixing bowl, whisk together the rice flour, sugar, baking powder, baking soda, and salt until well combined.

2. **Combine Wet Ingredients:**

   - In a separate bowl, whisk together the buttermilk, egg, melted butter (or oil), and vanilla extract.

3. **Mix Batter:**

   - Pour the wet ingredients into the dry ingredients and stir until just combined. Be cautious not to overmix; a few lumps are okay. Let the batter rest for a couple of

minutes to allow the rice
flour to absorb the liquid.

4. **Preheat Griddle or Pan:**

   - Preheat a griddle or non-
     stick pan over medium
     heat. Add a small amount
     of butter or oil to prevent
     sticking.

5. **Cook Pancakes:**

   - Pour 1/4 cup portions of
     batter onto the griddle for
     each pancake. Cook until
     bubbles form on the
     surface, then flip and
     cook the other side until
     golden brown.

6. **Serve Warm:**

   - Transfer the cooked
     pancakes to a plate and
     keep warm. Repeat the

process until all the
batter is used.

7. **Top and Enjoy:**

- Serve the gluten-free
  pancakes warm with
  your favorite toppings,
  such as maple syrup,
  fresh fruit, or whipped
  cream.

These gluten-free pancakes made with rice flour are not only delicious but also versatile. Feel free to add mix-ins like blueberries, chocolate chips, or chopped nuts for an extra flavor boost. Enjoy a delightful and gluten-free breakfast with this easy pancake recipe.

7.2 Crispy Rice Flour Cookies

These crispy rice flour cookies are gluten-free and delightful, offering a satisfying crunch with every bite. Perfect for any occasion, these cookies are easy to make and sure to be a hit.

Ingredients:

- 1 cup rice flour

- 1/2 cup butter, softened

- 1/2 cup sugar

- 1 teaspoon vanilla extract

- 1/4 teaspoon salt

- 1/2 cup rice cereal (crushed)

- Optional: Chocolate chips, chopped nuts, or dried fruit for added flavor

Instructions:

1. **Preheat Oven:**

   - Preheat your oven to
     350°F (175°C) and line a
     baking sheet with
     parchment paper.

2. **Cream Butter and Sugar:**

   - In a mixing bowl, cream
     together the softened
     butter and sugar until
     light and fluffy.

3. **Add Vanilla Extract:**

   - Mix in the vanilla
     extract, ensuring it's well
     incorporated.

4. **Combine Dry Ingredients:**

   - In a separate bowl, whisk
     together the rice flour
     and salt.

5. **Combine Wet and Dry Ingredients:**

- Gradually add the dry ingredients to the wet ingredients, mixing until a smooth dough forms.

6. **Fold in Rice Cereal:**

- Gently fold in the crushed rice cereal until evenly distributed throughout the cookie dough. If desired, add optional mix-ins like chocolate chips, nuts, or dried fruit.

7. **Shape Cookies:**

- Scoop tablespoon-sized portions of dough and place them on the prepared baking sheet.

Flatten each cookie
slightly with the back of
a spoon.

8. **Bake:**

   - Bake in the preheated
     oven for 10-12 minutes
     or until the edges are
     golden brown.

9. **Cool and Enjoy:**

   - Allow the cookies to cool
     on the baking sheet for a
     few minutes before
     transferring them to a
     wire rack to cool
     completely. Enjoy the
     crispy goodness!

These rice flour cookies offer a
delightful texture and can be
customized with your favorite
additions. Whether enjoyed with a

cup of tea or as a sweet treat on their own, these cookies are a gluten-free delight.

7.3 Rice Flour Bread

Savor the goodness of homemade gluten-free bread with this rice flour bread recipe. Soft and versatile, this bread is perfect for sandwiches, toast, or as a side to your favorite meals.

Ingredients:

- 2 cups rice flour

- 1 cup potato starch

- 1/2 cup tapioca flour

- 1 tablespoon active dry yeast

- 1 tablespoon sugar

- 1 1/2 teaspoons xanthan gum

- 1 teaspoon salt

- 1 1/4 cups warm water (110°F/43°C)

- 3 large eggs

- 1/4 cup vegetable oil

- 1 tablespoon apple cider vinegar

Instructions:

1. **Activate Yeast:**

   - In a small bowl, combine the warm water, sugar, and yeast. Let it sit for 5-10 minutes until frothy.

2. **Prepare Dry Ingredients:**

   - In a large mixing bowl, whisk together the rice flour, potato starch,

tapioca flour, xanthan
gum, and salt.

3. **Mix Wet Ingredients:**

- In a separate bowl, beat
  the eggs and add the
  vegetable oil and apple
  cider vinegar. Mix well.

4. **Combine and Mix:**

- Pour the activated yeast
  mixture into the dry
  ingredients, followed by
  the wet ingredients. Mix
  until well combined.

5. **Transfer to Pan:**

- Grease a 9x5-inch loaf
  pan. Transfer the bread
  batter into the pan and
  smooth the top with a
  spatula.

6. **Rise:**

- Cover the pan with a
  clean kitchen towel and
  let the bread rise in a
  warm place for about 1
  hour, or until it doubles
  in size.

7. **Preheat Oven:**

- Preheat the oven to
  375°F (190°C).

8. **Bake:**

- Bake the bread in the
  preheated oven for 25-30
  minutes, or until golden
  brown and the internal
  temperature reaches
  200°F (93°C).

9. **Cool and Slice:**

- Allow the bread to cool
  in the pan for 10 minutes
  before transferring it to a
  wire rack to cool
  completely. Slice and
  enjoy!

This rice flour bread is a fantastic gluten-free alternative, providing a soft and moist texture that makes it suitable for various uses. Whether toasted with butter or used for sandwiches, it's a delicious and versatile addition to your gluten-free baking repertoire.

CHAPTER 8

Health Considerations

8.1 Gluten-Free Diet

A gluten-free diet involves avoiding foods that contain gluten—a protein found in wheat, barley, rye, and their derivatives. For individuals with celiac disease, gluten sensitivity, or wheat allergy, adhering to a gluten-free diet is crucial. Rice flour plays a significant role in gluten-free cooking, providing a versatile and widely used alternative to traditional wheat flour. Here are some health considerations related to a gluten-free diet:

1. **Celiac Disease:**

   - Celiac disease is an autoimmune disorder where the ingestion of gluten leads to damage in the small intestine. Individuals with celiac disease must strictly adhere to a gluten-free diet to manage symptoms and prevent long-term complications.

2. **Non-Celiac Gluten Sensitivity:**

- Some people experience symptoms similar to those of celiac disease when consuming gluten but do not have the autoimmune response seen in celiac disease. This condition is known as non-celiac gluten sensitivity. A gluten-free diet may be recommended to manage symptoms.

3. **Wheat Allergy:**

- Wheat allergy is an allergic reaction to proteins found in wheat, including but not limited to gluten. Those with a wheat allergy need to avoid wheat-containing products, making gluten-free alternatives, such as rice flour, essential in their diet.

4. **Inflammatory Bowel Diseases:**

   - Individuals with inflammatory bowel diseases (such as Crohn's disease or ulcerative colitis) may find relief from symptoms by adopting a gluten-free diet. However, it's important to consult with a healthcare professional for personalized dietary advice.

5. **Autism Spectrum Disorders:**

   - Some individuals with autism spectrum disorders (ASD) may

follow a gluten-free diet, as some parents and caregivers believe it can improve certain behaviors. However, scientific evidence on the effectiveness of a gluten-free diet for ASD is limited, and consultation with healthcare providers is recommended.

6. **Gluten-Free Diet Challenges:**

- Following a gluten-free diet can be challenging due to the ubiquity of gluten in many processed foods. It requires careful label reading and attention to cross-contamination in both home cooking and when dining out.

7. **Nutritional Considerations:**

- While rice flour is a common and versatile gluten-free alternative, it's essential to pay attention to the nutritional aspects of a gluten-free diet. Some gluten-free products may lack certain nutrients found in fortified wheat products, such as B vitamins and iron. A well-balanced and varied diet is crucial.

8. **Gluten-Free Whole Foods:**

- Emphasizing naturally gluten-free whole foods, such as fruits, vegetables, lean proteins, dairy, and gluten-free grains like

rice, quinoa, and corn,
can contribute to a
nutrient-rich gluten-free
diet.

Individuals considering or following a gluten-free diet should seek guidance from healthcare professionals or registered dietitians to ensure that their nutritional needs are met. Additionally, for those with specific medical conditions such as celiac disease, proper diagnosis and ongoing medical supervision are essential for effective management and overall well-being.

8.2 Nutritional Benefits and Considerations of Rice Flour

Rice flour, a gluten-free alternative to traditional wheat flour, offers several nutritional benefits and considerations. Understanding its nutritional profile can help individuals make informed choices when incorporating it into their diets.

Nutritional Benefits:

1. **Gluten-Free Option:** Rice flour is naturally gluten-free, making it a suitable choice for individuals with celiac disease, gluten sensitivity, or those following a gluten-free diet.

2. **Rich in Carbohydrates:** Rice flour is a good source of carbohydrates, providing

energy for the body. It serves as a staple in many gluten-free recipes, including bread, pancakes, and cookies.

3. **Low in Fat:** Rice flour is naturally low in fat, making it a versatile ingredient for various culinary applications without significantly contributing to the overall fat content of a dish.

4. **Diverse Varieties:** Different types of rice flour exist, including white rice flour, brown rice flour, and sweet rice flour (glutinous rice flour). Each variety offers distinct flavors and nutritional nuances, allowing for diverse applications in cooking and baking.

5. **Rich in Essential Nutrients:**
   While rice flour is not as
   nutritionally dense as whole
   grains, it does provide essential
   nutrients such as manganese,
   magnesium, phosphorus, and
   niacin.

Considerations:

1. **Lower Fiber Content:**
   Compared to whole grains, rice
   flour tends to be lower in
   dietary fiber, which is crucial
   for digestive health. Individuals
   on a gluten-free diet should
   ensure they get sufficient fiber
   from other sources like fruits,
   vegetables, and gluten-free
   whole grains.

2. **Potential Nutrient Variations:**
   The nutritional content of rice
   flour can vary depending on the

type of rice used and the milling process. Brown rice flour retains more nutrients, including fiber and vitamins, compared to white rice flour, which is more refined.

3. **Glycemic Impact:** Rice flour may have a higher glycemic index compared to some other gluten-free flours, potentially leading to a quicker rise in blood sugar levels. Combining rice flour with other flours, incorporating fiber-rich ingredients, and managing portion sizes can help mitigate this effect.

4. **Balanced Diet:** While rice flour can be part of a balanced gluten-free diet, it's essential to include a variety of nutrient-dense foods to ensure

comprehensive nutritional intake. This includes incorporating a mix of fruits, vegetables, lean proteins, and other gluten-free grains.

5. **Consider Fortified Varieties:** Some commercially available rice flours may be fortified with additional nutrients, such as B vitamins and iron, to enhance their nutritional value. Checking product labels can help individuals make choices aligned with their nutritional goals.

Individuals with specific dietary considerations or medical conditions should consult with healthcare professionals or registered dietitians for personalized advice. While rice flour offers valuable options for gluten-free cooking and baking, a

well-rounded and diverse diet is key
to meeting overall nutritional needs.

9 7 9 8 8 6 8 1 4 1 0 7 2